Discover! 4

How to Stay Healthy

Julie Penn

Contents

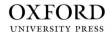

OXFORD
UNIVERSITY PRESS

OXFORD
UNIVERSITY PRESS

Great Clarendon Street, Oxford OX2 6DP

Oxford University Press is a department of the University of Oxford. It furthers the University's objective of excellence in research, scholarship, and education by publishing worldwide in

Oxford New York

Auckland Cape Town Dar es Salaam Hong Kong Karachi Kuala Lumpur Madrid Melbourne Mexico City Nairobi New Delhi Shanghai Taipei Toronto

With offices in

Argentina Austria Brazil Chile Czech Republic France Greece Guatemala Hungary Italy Japan Poland Portugal Singapore South Korea Switzerland Thailand Turkey Ukraine Vietnam

OXFORD and OXFORD ENGLISH are registered trade marks of Oxford University Press in the UK and in certain other countries

© Oxford University Press 2011

The moral rights of the author have been asserted

Database right Oxford University Press (maker)

First published 2011

2017

13

No unauthorized photocopying

ISBN: 978 0 19 464445 7

An Audio Pack containing this book and an Audio download is also available, ISBN: 978 0 19 402204 0

This book is also available as an e-Book, ISBN: 978 0 19 410890 4.

An accompanying Activity Book is also available, ISBN: 978 0 19 464455 6

Printed in China

This book is printed on paper from certified and well-managed sources.

ACKNOWLEDGEMENTS

Illustrations by: Kelly Kennedy pp.5, 7, 13; Ian Moores Graphics pp.6, 16, 26, 36, 42; Dusan Pavlic/Beehive Illustration pp.28, 38, 40, 46-47; Alan Rowe pp.28, 42, 46-47; Mark Ruffle p.30.

The Publishers would also like to thank the following for their kind permission to reproduce photographs and other copyright material: Alamy pp.5 (Everyday Images), 10 (allOver photography/ Japanese food), 11 (Tim Hill/soup), 19 (cycling at night); Corbis p.4, (Jim Sugar), 10 (Karen Kasmauski/girl); Getty Images pp.14 (Chris Clinton/Taxi), 15 (Mickey Bushell of Great Britain competes in Men's 200m T53 heats, London 2012 Paralympic Games/Gareth Copley), 17 (Alexander Hubrich/Stone/sprinters); Oxford University Press pp.3, 8-9, 13 (girl brushing teeth), 17 (sea swimming), 18, 19 (girl drinking), 20 (mountain biking), 21, 22 , 23; Photolibrary pp.11 (Katja Kreder/bread and salad), 20 (Mark Thayer/ Index Stock Imagery/rollerblading); Science Photo Library pp.12 (Coneyl Jay), 13 (CNRI/decayed tooth).

With thanks to Ann Fullick for science checking

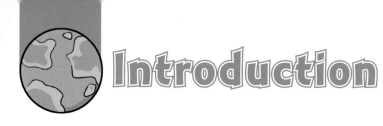

Introduction

Do you know how to stay healthy? Think about the exercise that you do and the food that you eat. Exercise and the right food help you to live longer.

Which of these types of exercise do you do?
When do you do exercise?

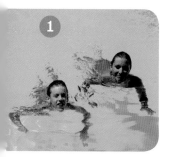

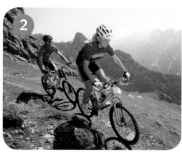

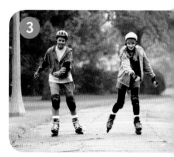

Which of this food do you eat?
How much water do you drink every day?

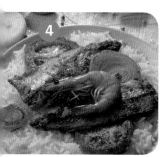

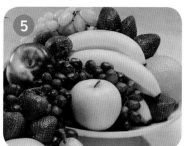

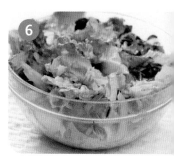

Now read and discover more about how to stay healthy!

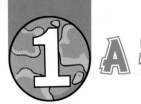

A Healthy Life

For a healthy life, you need to protect your body. Your body needs exercise and the right food. Most people can do some exercise. Some people have disabilities, but they can do exercise, too. You don't need lots of time or equipment to do exercise. Things that you do every day can help you to stay healthy, like walking to the supermarket or to school.

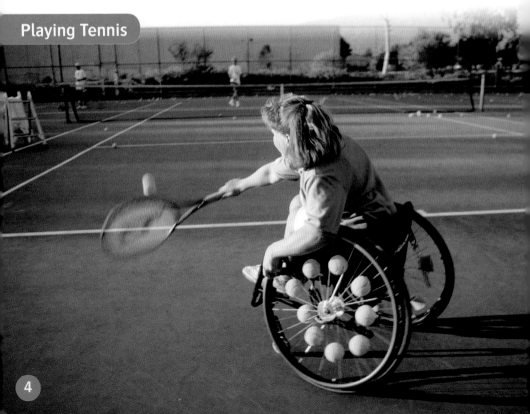

Playing Tennis

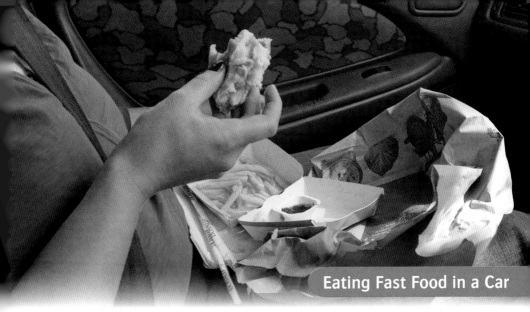

Eating Fast Food in a Car

Some people need medicines every day to stay healthy. A long time ago, there were no medicines for sick people. Today, there are medicines, but there's a new problem – people are getting fatter. Many people eat too much. A lot of food today is unhealthy, for example, fast food. Many people don't do much exercise outdoors. They watch television, use the computer, and play computer games. They travel by car a lot, too.

Discover! People around the world eat about 11 million metric tons of French fries every year.

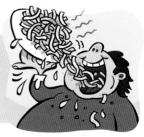

→ Go to pages 24–25 for activities.

5

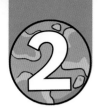

Inside Your Body

Inside your body, there are many different parts. They help you to stay healthy. Do you know what they do?

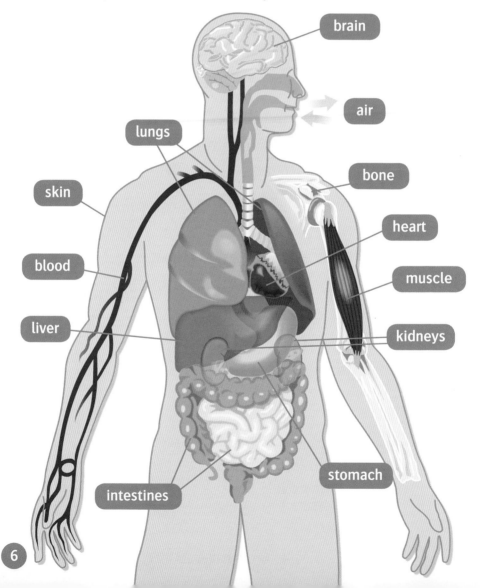

brain

air

lungs

bone

skin

heart

blood

muscle

liver

kidneys

intestines

stomach

Your brain makes the different parts of your body work well. Your lungs help you to breathe. Air goes in and out of your lungs when you breathe. This gives you the oxygen that you need. Your heart moves blood around your body. The blood takes oxygen and food to the different parts of your body.

Your bones are very strong and they support your body. They also protect important parts of your body, like the brain and heart. Your muscles help your body to move. Your skin protects your body. It also helps to keep your body at the right temperature.

Your stomach and intestines break down the food that you eat, so that your body can use the food. Your liver and kidneys take away the things that your body doesn't need.

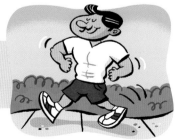

Discover! You use about 200 different muscles to walk!

→ Go to pages 26–27 for activities.

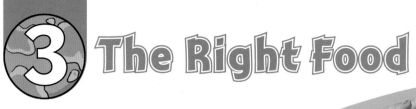

The Right Food

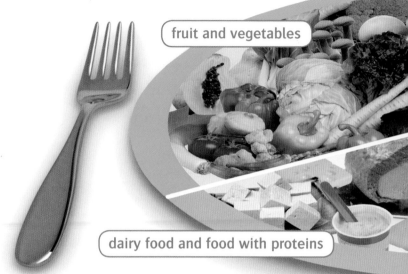

fruit and vegetables

dairy food and food with proteins

You need to eat the right food. Carbohydrates give your body energy. Fiber helps to move food through your stomach and intestines. Brown bread and brown rice have lots of fiber. Fruit and vegetables also have fiber, and vitamins that help you to stay healthy.

Proteins help your muscles to grow. Meat, fish, and eggs have proteins. Dairy food like milk, yogurt, and cheese have proteins, fat, and calcium. You need calcium for healthy bones. You need iron for healthy blood. Meat, eggs, and green vegetables have iron.

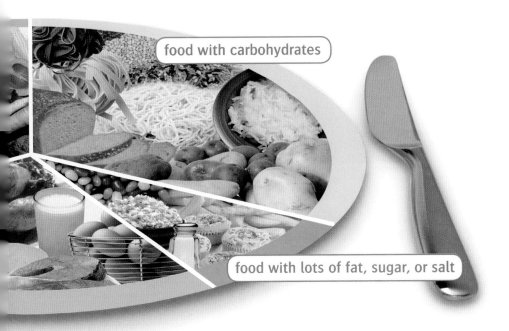

food with carbohydrates

food with lots of fat, sugar, or salt

This plate shows how much of each type of food you should eat. Eat lots of fruit and vegetables, and food with proteins and carbohydrates. Don't eat too much food with sugar, fat, and salt. You need a little fat to stay healthy, but too much fat can make you fat! Too much sugar and salt is unhealthy, too. Sugar is also bad for your teeth.

Discover!

You should drink about eight glasses of water every day.

→ Go to pages 28–29 for activities.

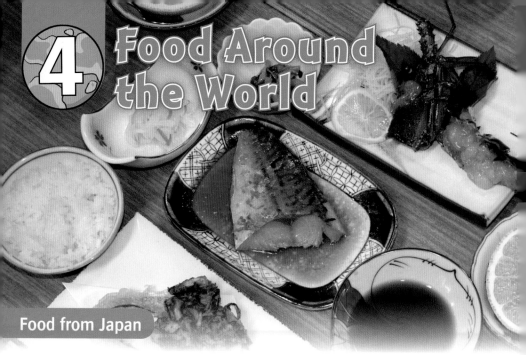

4 Food Around the World

Food from Japan

Around the world, people eat different food to stay healthy. What healthy food around the world do you know?

In Japan, people eat lots of rice, vegetables, and fish. This food has lots of fiber and vitamins. It doesn't have much fat.

Discover!

Many people in Asia use chopsticks to cook and eat food. Chopsticks were invented in China about 5,000 years ago.

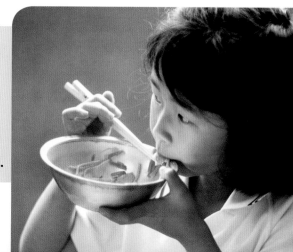

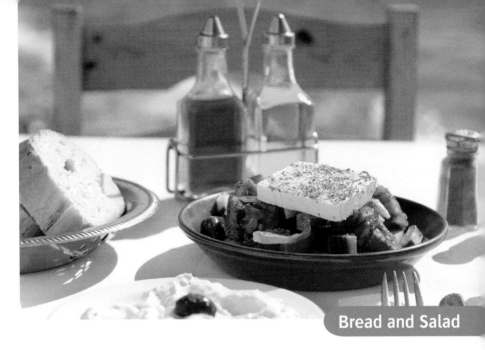

Bread and Salad

In countries near the Mediterranean Sea, people eat lots of bread, salad, and fruit. They use olive oil and tomatoes for making salads and for cooking. Scientists think that olive oil and tomatoes help people to stay healthy.

Quinoa Soup

In Peru and Bolivia, people eat lots of fruit and vegetables. Some people eat rice or quinoa seeds with meat and potatoes. Quinoa has lots of proteins, fiber, and iron.

quinoa

→ Go to pages 30–31 for activites.

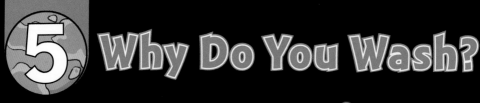

5 Why Do You Wash?

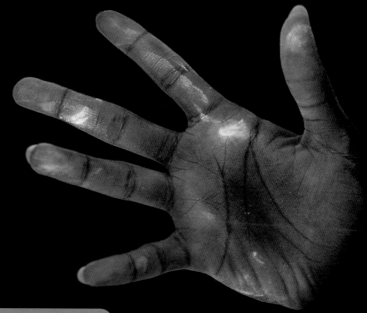

Microbes on a Hand

Did you know that millions of microbes live on your hands? Microbes are very, very small living things – you can't see them! Some microbes aren't dangerous, but some can make you sick.

Remember to wash your hands. It's important to wash away the microbes after you go to the toilet, and after you touch dirty things. Wash your hands before you touch food, too.

Meat that's not cooked has dangerous microbes. Wash your hands after you touch meat that's not cooked, and cook meat well.

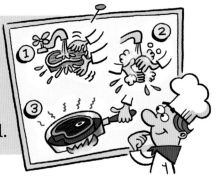

It's important to brush your teeth every day. When you eat food with sugar, the microbes on your teeth also eat the sugar. This can damage your teeth and make your teeth unhealthy.

To keep your teeth healthy, brush them with toothpaste to wash away the microbes. Go to the dentist every year, and don't eat too much food with sugar.

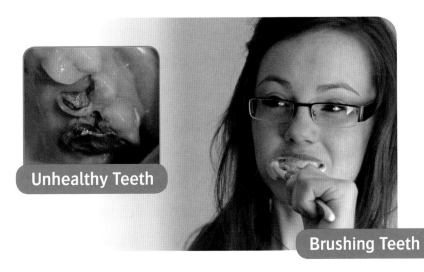

Unhealthy Teeth

Brushing Teeth

Go to pages 32–33 for activities.

6 Exercise for Everyone

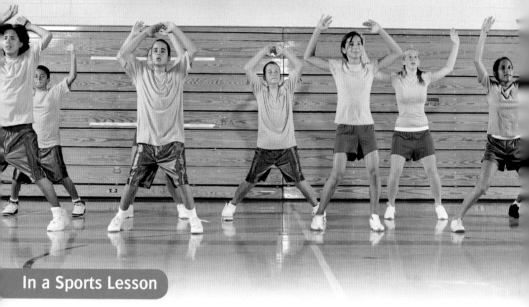

In a Sports Lesson

Why is exercise good? It helps to make your bones and muscles stronger. It also protects you from health problems. It makes you feel good, and it even helps you to work better at school!

Everyone needs to do exercise to stay healthy. Exercise isn't only for young, healthy people. Older people and people with health problems or disabilities need exercise, too. Everyone can find an exercise that they can do. What exercise do you do?

It's good to do some exercise every day, but you don't need to go to the sports center all the time. You can play sports in the park and help with jobs at home. Swimming is a good exercise, and most people can do it.

Many people with disabilities can do team sports and athletics, too. Some of the world's most amazing sports people have disabilities.

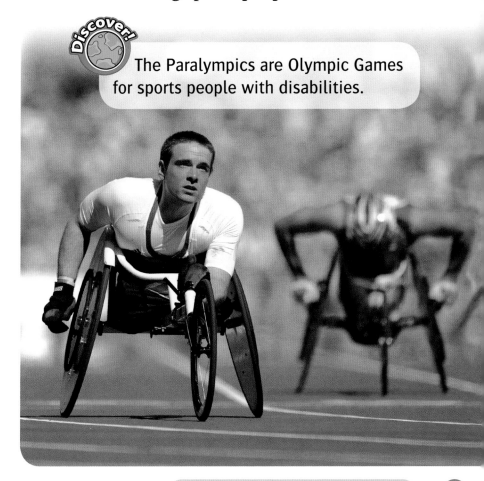

Discover!

The Paralympics are Olympic Games for sports people with disabilities.

→ Go to pages 34–35 for activities.

7 Exercise and Your Body

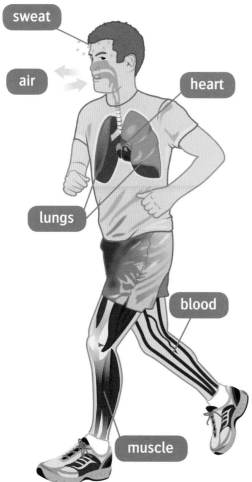

sweat

air

heart

lungs

blood

muscle

When you do exercise, you breathe faster. Your lungs take in more air to give your body more oxygen. Your heart beats faster, so it moves blood to your muscles faster. The blood takes oxygen and food for the muscles to use.

Your body gets hotter when you do exercise. Your skin feels hot, and you make water called sweat. When your skin dries, you cool down.

Discover!

Most people make more than 1 liter of sweat in one hour of exercise. That's one big bottle of water!

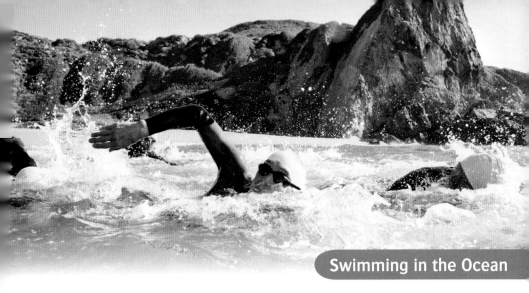

Swimming in the Ocean

Your muscles need oxygen to work well for a long time. When you walk, jog, cycle, or swim, you breathe faster to give your muscles the oxygen that they need. This exercise makes you more healthy.

Running Fast

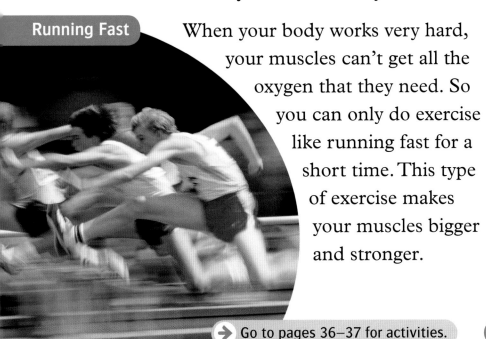

When your body works very hard, your muscles can't get all the oxygen that they need. So you can only do exercise like running fast for a short time. This type of exercise makes your muscles bigger and stronger.

Go to pages 36–37 for activities.

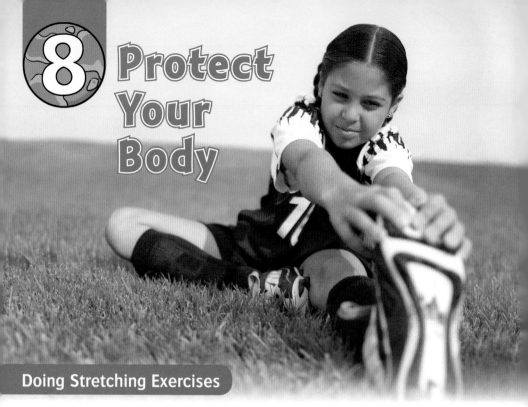

8 Protect Your Body

Doing Stretching Exercises

Before you start your exercise, it's good to warm up your muscles, so that you don't damage them. When you warm up your muscles, they move more easily. Walk, jog, or skip for a few minutes. You should also do some stretching exercises. These help you to move your arms and legs easily.

Think about how you breathe when you do exercise. When you don't breathe well, your brain and muscles don't get all the oxygen that they need. You should breathe slowly and deeply.

After you finish your exercise, it's good to cool down your muscles, so that they don't get sore. Run slowly or walk for a few minutes. Then do more stretching exercises. You also need to put back the water that you lose in your sweat, so it's important to drink after you do exercise.

Stay safe when you do exercise. Use the right equipment to protect your head and body. When you are doing exercise outdoors in the dark, people need to see you. Wear bright clothes and use lights when you cycle.

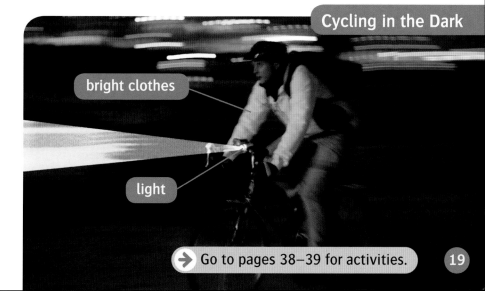

Cycling in the Dark

bright clothes

light

Go to pages 38–39 for activities.

9 Time Outdoors

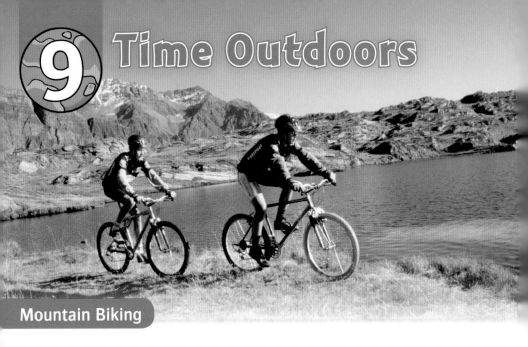

Mountain Biking

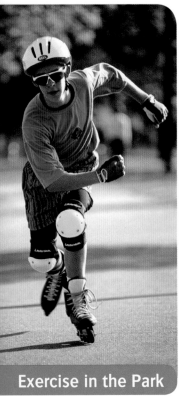

Exercise in the Park

It's good to spend time outdoors. Scientists think that it makes you feel happier and it helps you to stay healthy.

When you are outdoors, it's easy to do exercise and have fun at the same time. Many people do team sports at school. Cycling and walking are good exercise, too. Some people do exciting adventure sports in the mountains, like climbing or mountain biking. What sports do you do outdoors?

You need to spend some time outdoors because your skin uses the sun to make Vitamin D. Vitamin D is important for healthy teeth and bones. Remember to wear suncream because the sun can also damage your skin. Wear sunglasses to protect your eyes.

These people are cleaning the countryside. They are picking up waste. It's a good way to protect our planet and to stay healthy at the same time!

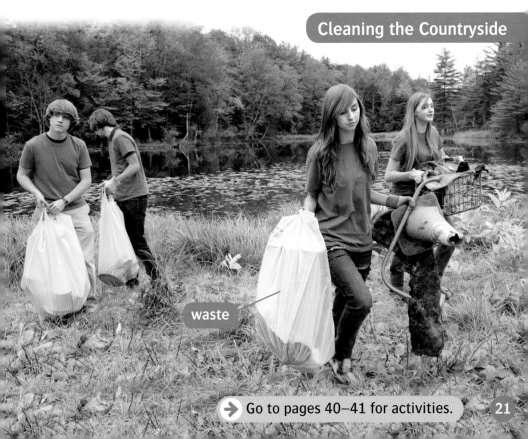

Cleaning the Countryside

waste

Go to pages 40–41 for activities.

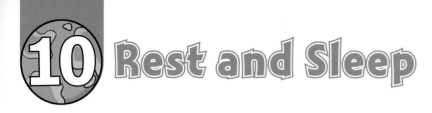

10 Rest and Sleep

It's very important to rest. When you do exercise, small pieces of protein in your muscles break. Your body needs time to repair your muscles, and to make them bigger. Don't make your body work too hard. When you do lots of exercise, it's important to rest the next day.

Some types of exercise help you to rest. There are yoga and tai chi exercises that teach people how to rest.

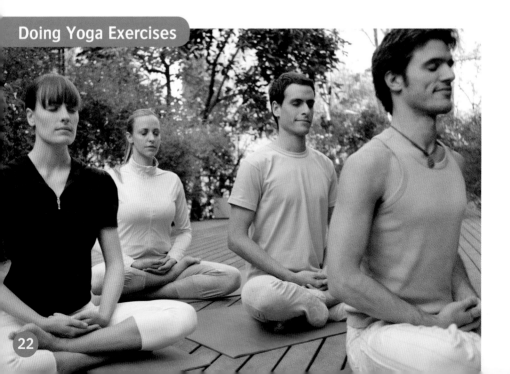

Doing Yoga Exercises

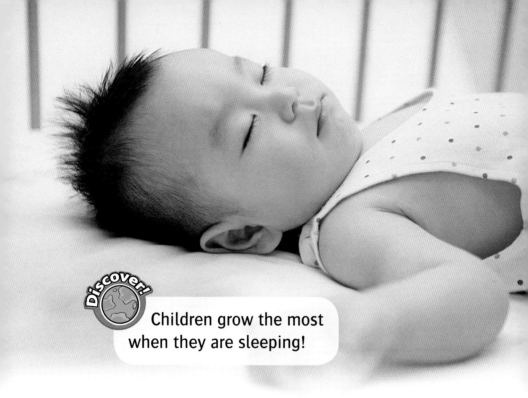

Discover! Children grow the most when they are sleeping!

It's also important to sleep well. Most people sleep between six and eight hours every night. Children need to sleep more than nine hours every night. You need to sleep so that your brain can rest. When you don't sleep well, your brain can't work well, and you feel tired and unhappy.

Remember, you feel good and stay healthy when you do the right things – you should eat well, do exercise, and have lots of sleep.

→ Go to pages 42–43 for activities.

① A Healthy Life

← Read pages 4–5.

1 Find the words.

bodytehealthyinmedicinesarexercisenifastfood

1 __body__ 2 _____ 3 _____

4 _____ 5 _____ 6 _____

2 Complete the sentences.

outdoors healthy travel ~~medicines~~
exercise disabilities body

1 Today there are __medicines__ for sick people.

2 People don't do much exercise _____ .

3 Some people have _____ .

4 You need to protect your _____ .

5 You don't need lots of time or equipment to do

_____ .

6 Walking to the supermarket can help you to stay

_____ .

7 People _____ by car a lot.

3 Write true or false.

1 People are getting fatter.   _true_

2 Fast food is healthy.   _____

3 Many people don't do much
exercise outdoors.   _____

4 Some people need medicines
every day to stay healthy.   _____

5 Most people can do exercise.   _____

6 Watching television helps you
to stay healthy.   _____

4 Answer the questions.

1 Do you walk to school or to the supermarket?

_____

2 Do you usually travel by car?

_____

3 Do you do exercise outdoors?

_____

4 Do you watch lots of television?

_____

5 Do you use the computer a lot?

_____

6 Do you eat lots of French fries?

_____

② Inside Your Body

← Read pages 6–7.

1 Write the words.

intestines stomach ~~brain~~
bone skin kidneys liver
muscle heart lungs

1 ___brain___
2 _____
3 _____
4 _____
5 _____
6 _____
7 _____
8 _____
9 _____
10 _____

2 Match.

1 It moves blood around your body.

2 It breaks down the food that you eat.

3 It makes different parts of your body work well.

4 It protects your body.

5 They support your body.

6 They help you to breathe.

lungs

brain

bones

heart

stomach

skin

3 Complete the sentences.

kidneys bones move blood
liver temperature breathe

1 Your _____ takes oxygen and food to different parts of your body.

2 Air goes in and out of your lungs when you _____.

3 Your _____ protect important parts of your body.

4 Your _____ and _____ take away the things that your body doesn't need.

5 Your skin helps to keep your body at the right _____.

6 Your muscles help your body to _____.

4 Write *true* or *false*.

1 Your brain makes the other parts of your body work well. _____

2 Your bones are very strong. _____

3 Your skin supports your body. _____

4 Your kidneys help your body to move. _____

5 Your stomach and intestines break down food so that your body can use it. _____

6 You use 20 different muscles to walk. _____

③ The Right Food

← Read pages 8–9.

1 Write the words.

bread   rice   fish   ~~fruit~~   vegetables   milk

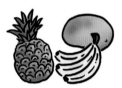

1 ___fruit___

2 _____

3 _____

4 _____

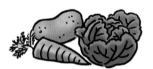

5 _____

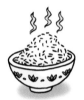

6 _____

2 Complete the chart.

~~bread~~   fish   meat   fruit   eggs   vegetables

Carbohydrates	Proteins	Vitamins
bread		

3 Complete the sentences.

sugar vitamins proteins fiber calcium fat

1 Meat, fish, and eggs have lots of _____ .

2 Too much fat can make you _____ .

3 Too much _____ is bad for your teeth.

4 Milk, yogurt, and cheese have _____ .

5 Fruit and vegetables have lots of _____ .

6 Brown bread and brown rice have lots of

_____ .

4 Match. Then write the sentences.

Carbohydrates

Fiber helps food to move

Proteins help

You need calcium

Too much fat, sugar, and salt

your muscles to grow.

through your stomach and intestines.

is unhealthy.

give your body energy.

for healthy bones.

1 _Carbohydrates give your body energy._

2 _____

3 _____

4 _____

5 _____

4 Food Around the World

← Read pages 10–11.

1 Complete the map.

Bolivia   China   ~~Peru~~   Japan   Mediterranean Sea

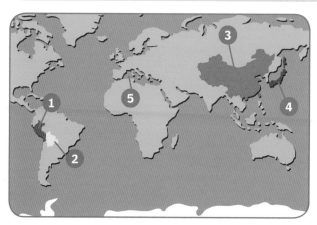

1 _____Peru_____

2 _____

3 _____

4 _____

5 _____

2 Find and write the food words.

o	l	i	v	e	o	i	l
l	a	v	e	g	e	t	i
i	s	a	g	i	c	e	s
r	i	c	e	m	b	o	a
o	f	o	t	e	r	a	l
f	r	u	a	s	m	d	a
m	u	o	b	r	e	a	d
r	i	c	l	o	a	l	a
s	t	t	e	l	t	a	d
a	f	i	s	h	a	l	s

1 fruit

2 v

3 s

4 r

5 f

6 m

7 b

8 o

3 Complete the sentences.

fat iron rice tomatoes salad chopsticks quinoa

1 In Japan, people eat lots of _____ .

2 Food in Japan doesn't have much _____ .

3 In countries near the Mediterranean Sea, people eat lots of bread, _____ , and fruit.

4 In Peru and Bolivia, some people eat rice or _____ with meat and potatoes.

5 In Asia, many people use _____ to eat food.

6 Scientists think that _____ can help you to stay healthy.

7 Quinoa has lots of proteins, fiber, and _____ .

4 Answer the questions.

1 What is the most popular food in your country?

_____

_____

2 Which food from your country is healthy?

_____

3 Which food from your country is unhealthy?

_____

5 Why Do You Wash?

1 Complete the poster.

food   meat   ~~Millions~~   toilet   sick   dirty

Did you know ...?

___Millions___ of microbes live on your hands!

Microbes can make you _____ .

Always wash your hands ...

before you touch _____ .

after you go to the _____ .

after you touch _____ things.

after you touch _____ that's not cooked.

2 Circle the correct words.

1 The microbes **on your hands** / **in your mouth** can damage your teeth.

2 Brush your teeth to wash away the **toothpaste** / **microbes**.

3 To keep your teeth healthy, go to the **dentist** / **doctor**.

4 Don't eat too much food with **vitamins** / **sugar**.

3 Write true or false.

1 All microbes are dangerous. _____

2 Some microbes can make you sick. _____

3 Meat that is not cooked
has dangerous microbes. _____

4 It's important to keep your
teeth clean. _____

5 When you eat food with sugar,
the microbes in your mouth
eat the sugar, too. _____

4 Answer the questions.

1 How many microbes live on your hands?

_____

2 What should you do before you touch food?

_____

3 What happens when you eat food with sugar?

_____

4 Why do you clean your teeth?

_____

5 What else can you do to keep your teeth healthy?

_____

6 Exercise For Everyone

← Read pages 14–15.

1 Complete the sentences.

good   healthy   problems   bones   work   muscles

Why is exercise good for you?

1 It helps to make your _____ and _____ stronger.

2 It protects you from health _____.

3 It makes you feel _____.

4 It helps you to _____ better at school.

5 It helps you to stay _____.

2 Match.

1 Everyone needs to do exercise

2 Exercise isn't only for

3 You need to do

4 Swimming is a good exercise,

5 Many people with disabilities

6 You don't have to

some exercise every day.

and most people can do it.

go to the sports center every day.

to stay healthy.

can do team sports and athletics.

young, healthy people.

3 Order the words.

1 exercise / healthy. / stay / do / needs / Everyone / to / to

Everyone needs to do exercise to stay healthy.

2 health problems. / Exercise / you / protects / from

_____

3 only / young / for / Exercise / people. / isn't

_____

4 good / a / Swimming / exercise. / is

_____

5 sports / the / You / in / play / park. / can

_____

6 helps / you / school. / better / at / Exercise / work / to

_____

4 Answer the questions.

1 What types of exercise do you do?

_____

2 What is your favorite type of exercise?

_____

3 How much exercise do you do every week?

_____

7 Exercise and Your Body

← Read pages 16–17.

1 Find and write the words.

uplungsfobreatheheartenbloodovfoodresweatuy

1 _____ 2 _____ 3 _____

4 _____ 5 _____ 6 _____

2 Complete the sentences.

> blood   cool down   breathe   heart   skin   lungs

1 When you do exercise,
you _____ faster.

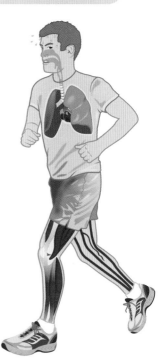

2 Your _____ take in
more air.

3 Your _____ beats faster.

4 Your _____ takes
oxygen and food to your
muscles.

5 Your _____ feels hot.

6 You make sweat. When your
skin dries, you _____ .

3 Circle the correct words.

1 Your muscles **need** / **don't need** oxygen to work well for a long time.

2 When you swim, you breathe **faster** / **slower**.

3 Swimming makes you **fatter** / **more healthy**.

4 When your body works very hard, your muscles **can** / **can't** get all the oxygen that they need.

5 You can only run fast for a **long** / **short** time.

6 Running fast makes your muscles **bigger** / **smaller**.

4 Answer the questions.

1 Why do you breathe faster when you do exercise?

_____

2 What does sweat do?

_____

3 What do your muscles need to work for a long time?

_____

4 What happens when your body works very hard?

_____

5 What exercises can you do for a long time?

_____

6 What exercise can you only do for a short time?

_____

8 Protect Your Body

← Read pages 18–19.

1 Write the words.

skip jog walk stretch

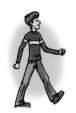

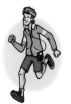
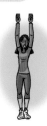

1 _____   2 _____   3 _____   4 _____

2 Complete the chart.

drink warm up your muscles do stretching exercises
cool down your muscles breathe slowly and deeply
do more stretching exercises

	What should you do?
Before Exercise	
When You Do Exercise	
After Exercise	

3 Complete the sentences.

cool down lights legs breathe
arms muscles equipment

1 When you warm up your _____ , they move
   more easily.

2 Stretching exercises help you to move your
   _____ and _____ easily.

3 Remember to _____ well when you do
   exercise.

4 After exercise you should _____ your
   muscles, so that they don't get sore.

5 Use the right _____ to protect your head
   and body.

6 Always use _____ when you cycle in the dark.

4 Find and write the words.

1 three ways to warm up your muscles

   _____

2 two ways to cool down your muscles

   _____

3 three ways to stay safe when you do exercise

   _____

9 Time Outdoors

← Read pages 20–21.

1 Write the words.

walking cycling adventure sports team sports

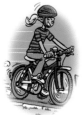 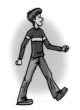 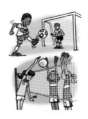 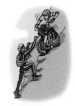

1 _____ 2 _____ 3 _____ 4 _____

_____   _____

2 Complete the sentences.

school sun happier bones teeth walking suncream

1 When you spend time outdoors it makes you feel
_____.

2 Many people do team sports at _____.

3 Cycling and _____ are good types of exercise.

4 Your skin uses the _____ to make Vitamin D.

5 Vitamin D is important for healthy _____ and
_____.

6 Wear _____ when you go outdoors.

3 Order the words.

1 time / It's / outdoors. / good / spend / to

_____

2 sports. /do / Some / exciting / people /adventure

_____

3 your / sun / skin. / can / The / damage

_____

4 wear / It's / suncream. / to / important

_____

5 do / outdoors? / do / sports / What / you

_____

6 uses / sun / to / Your / Vitamin D. / make / skin / the

_____

4 Answer the questions.

1 How much time do you spend time outdoors?

_____

2 Where do you go? What do you do?

_____

_____

_____

10 Rest and Sleep

← Read pages 22–23.

1 Complete the puzzle.

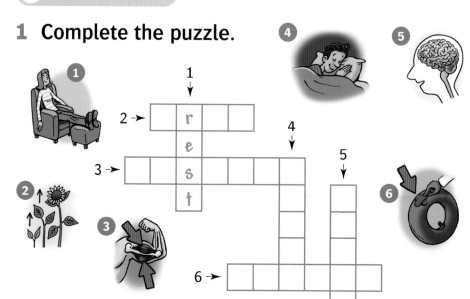

2 Write *true* or *false*.

1 Your body needs time to repair your muscles.

_____

2 You don't need to rest after you do lots of exercise.

_____

3 Some types of exercise help you to rest.

_____

4 Most people sleep between six and eight hours every night.

_____

5 Children need to sleep for more than ninety hours every night.

_____

3 Complete the sentences.

brain hard protein good repair healthy

1 When you do exercise, small pieces of _____ in your muscles break.

2 Your body needs time to _____ your muscles.

3 Don't make your body work too _____.

4 When you don't sleep well, your _____ can't work well.

5 You feel _____ and stay _____ when you do the right things.

4 Answer the questions.

1 What happens to your muscles when you do exercise?_____

_____

2 Why do you need sleep?

_____

3 How many hours do most people sleep?

_____

4 How many hours do you usually sleep?

_____

5 Do you do the right things to stay healthy?

_____

My Favorite Lunch

1 Complete the chart about your favorite lunch.

What is your favorite lunch? _____

What is in it?	None	Some	A Lot
Fat			
Sugar			
Salt			
Proteins			
Carbohydrates			
Fiber			
Vitamins			

2 Write about your favorite lunch. What is healthy? What is unhealthy?

_____

_____

_____

_____

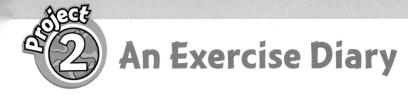

An Exercise Diary

1 Write what types of exercise you do in a week.

Monday	Friday
Tuesday	Saturday
Wednesday	
Thursday	Sunday

2 Look at your diary and complete the chart.

Questions	Score Yes = 1 point No = 0 points
Did you do lots of exercise?	
Did you do different types of exercise?	
Did you rest on some days?	
Total =	___/3

Picture Dictionary

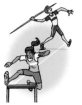
athletics

beat

breathe

children

clothes

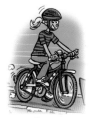
cycling

dangerous

deep

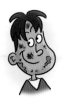
dirty

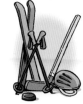
equipment

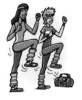
exercise

fat

food

French fries

fruit

glasses

grow

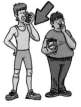
healthy

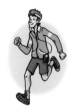
jog

meat